CHEST INFECTION

An essential book On how to treat chest infections

Dr Rowan Theo

Table of Contents

CHAPTER ONE

Identifying and Treating Chest Infections

What is a chest contamination?

A chest contamination is a form of breathing contamination that affects the decrease a part of your breathing tract.

Your decrease breathing tract consists of your windpipe, bronchi, and lungs.

The maximum common varieties of chest infections are bronchitis and pneumonia. Chest infections can variety everywhere from slight to intense.

What are the signs and symptoms of a chest contamination?

The signs and symptoms of a chest contamination can consist of:

• chesty cough (moist or phlegmy)

• wheezing

• coughing up yellow or inexperienced mucus

• feeling quick of breath

• soreness on your chest

• fever

• headache

• muscle aches and pains

• feeling worn-out or fatigued

What reasons a chest contamination?

A chest contamination may be resulting from a bacterial or viral contamination. The specific purpose will rely upon the form of contamination.

For example, bronchitis is frequently resulting from a virus, while maximum instances of pneumonia are bacterial in origin.

You can capture a chest contamination via way of means of breathing in the breathing droplets which might be generated while a person with an contamination coughs or sneezes.

That's due to the fact the breathing droplets convey the contamination.

Additionally, entering touch with a floor that's infected with the virus or micro organism, after which touching your mouth or face also can unfold the contamination.

You can be at an expanded chance for a chest contamination in case you:

• are elderly

• are pregnant

• are a toddler or younger infant

• smoke

- have a continual fitness circumstance, together with continual obstructive pulmonary disorder (COPD), bronchial allergies, or diabetes

- have a weakened immune machine, both from a circumstance such HIV, or from being the recipient of an organ transplant

When to are seeking assist from a healthcare provider

In a few instances, a chest contamination, together with acute bronchitis, will leave on its personal and also you won't must see a physician.

A pharmacist can be capin a position that will help you via way of means of recommending over-the-counter (OTC) decongestant medicines to assist loosen any mucus on your chest, with the intention to make it simpler to cough up.

You ought to usually visit see a physician for a chest contamination in case you:

• are over sixty five years old

• have a infant beneath five with signs and symptoms of a chest contamination

• are pregnant

- have a continual fitness circumstance or a weakened immune machine

• cough up blood or bloody mucus

- have signs and symptoms together with a fever or headache that receives worse

- have a cough that lasts longer than 3 weeks

- have brief breathing, ache on your chest, or shortness of breath

- sense dizzy, confused, or disoriented

In order to diagnose your circumstance, the physician will examine your signs and symptoms and carry out a bodily exam, in the course of which they'll use a stethoscope to concentrate in your coronary heart and lungs as you breathe.

The physician might also additionally take a chest X-ray to decide the vicinity and severity of your contamination.

They may additionally take a sputum or blood pattern to discover what's inflicting your contamination. If micro organism are inflicting your chest contamination, those assessments also can assist them determine which antibiotic to use.

CHAPTER TWO

How to deal with a chest contamination

If your chest contamination is resulting from a virus, antibiotics won't be effective. Instead, your remedy will consciousness on easing your signs and symptoms till you start to get higher.

If you've got a bacterial contamination, you'll be handled with antibiotics. In a slight case, you may take those at domestic in pill form.

If you've got a intense bacterial chest contamination, you could want to be handled with IV antibiotics in a medical institution.

Always take the whole direction of antibiotics, even in case you start to sense higher.

Home treatments for chest contamination

These domestic treatments might also additionally assist ease the signs and symptoms of your chest contamination. Try those hints:

• Take OTC medicines together with ibuprofen (Advil) or acetaminophen (Tylenol) to decrease your fever and assist relieve any aches and pains.

• Use OTC decongestants or expectorants to assist loosen mucus and make it simpler to cough up.

• Be certain to get masses of rest.

• Drink plenty of fluids. This maintains you hydrated and may loosen mucus, making it simpler to cough up.

• Avoid mendacity flat while sleeping. This can purpose mucus to settle on your chest. Use more pillows to raise your head and chest at night time.

• Use a humidifier or inhale steam vapor to assist relieve coughing.

• Have a heat drink of honey and lemon in case your throat is sore from an excessive amount of coughing.

• Avoid smoking, or being round secondhand smoke or different irritants.

• Stay far from cough suppression drugs. Coughing virtually lets you recover from your contamination via clearing mucus out of your lungs.

How lengthy does it take to get over a chest contamination?

Most chest contamination signs and symptoms commonly leave

inside 7 to ten days, despite the fact that a cough can last as long as 3 weeks.

See your physician in case your signs and symptoms haven't progressed or are becoming worse on this time.

What are feasible headaches from a chest contamination?

Sometimes, a case of bronchitis can cause pneumonia in a few individuals.

The feasible headaches from a chest contamination like pneumonia can consist of:

• micro organism on your bloodstream (sepsis)

• accumulation of fluid inside your lungs

• improvement of lung abscesses

How to save you a chest contamination

You can assist save you chest infections via way of means of following the hints below:

• Make certain your palms are clean, mainly earlier than consuming or touching your face or mouth.

• Eat a healthful properly-balanced diet. This can assist improve your immune machine and make you much less at risk of contamination.

• Get vaccinated. Chest infections can increase following an contamination together with influenza, for which there's a seasonal vaccine. You may additionally need to remember receiving the pneumococcal vaccine, which gives safety from pneumonia.

• Avoid smoking and publicity to secondhand smoke.

• Reduce the quantity of alcohol which you consume.

• If you're already ill, wash your palms often and make certain to cowl your mouth while you cough or sneeze. Dispose of any used tissues properly.

The outlook

Chest infections may be resulting from a viral or bacterial contamination on your decrease breathing tract. They can variety from slight to intense.

Many slight chest infections will clear up on their personal in approximately a week's time. A chest contamination that's resulting from micro organism will want to be handled with a direction of antibiotics.

Severe or complex chest infections might also additionally require remedy in a medical institution.

CHAPTER THREE

What approximately antibiotics?

Antibiotics are drugs used for infections resulting from germs (micro organism) and do not paintings on viruses. Unless you've got an extended-time period circumstance affecting your chest, your physician is not going to prescribe antibiotics except your signs and symptoms and exam advocate you could have pneumonia.

What can I do to deal with my chest contamination?

If you've got a chest contamination, you ought to:

• Have masses of rest.

• Drink plenty to save you your frame turning into missing in fluids (dehydrated) and to assist hold the mucus on your lungs skinny and simpler to cough up.

• Inhale steam vapour, possibly with brought menthol. This can assist to clean the mucus out of your chest. Never use warm water for a infant's cough, in case they get scalded via way of means of accident

• Avoid mendacity flat at night time to assist hold your chest clean of mucus and make it simpler to breathe.

• Take paracetamol, ibuprofen or aspirin to lessen excessive temperature and to ease any aches, pains and headaches. (Note: kids elderly much less than sixteen years ought to now no longer take aspirin.)

• If you smoke, you ought to try and forestall smoking for properly. Bronchitis, chest infections and severe lung sicknesses are extra common in smokers.

• If your throat is sore from coughing, you may relieve the

soreness with a heat drink of honey and lemon.

What approximately bloodless and cough drugs?

You should purchase many bloodless treatments and cough drugs at pharmacies. There is restrained proof of any gain from taking bloodless and cough treatments.

Infection of the huge airlines (bronchi) in the lungs (acute bronchitis) commonly clears with none headaches. Occasionally, the contamination travels to the lung tissue to purpose a severe lung contamination (pneumonia).

If you've got pneumonia and are properly sufficient to be taken care of at domestic, your outlook could be very properly. If you want to be taken care of in medical institution, the outlook remains commonly properly - however now no longer pretty as properly. The outlook is likewise now no longer as properly for those who additionally have lengthy-time period ailments together with lung disorder, coronary heart failure or diabetes.

When ought to you spot a physician?

Infection of the huge airlines (bronchi) in the lungs (acute bronchitis) commonly receives higher via way of means of itself, so there's frequently no want to peer a physician. If you've got bronchial allergies or COPD you ought to take your physician's recommendation. They might also additionally have given you guidelines approximately growing your inhaler medicinal drug or taking a 'rescue pack' of antibiotics and steroid capsules at the primary signal of an contamination. If now no longer, communicate with them for recommendation in case you increase signs and symptoms of a chest contamination.

There are some of signs and symptoms that suggest you ought to see a physician even in case you do now no longer have every other lung troubles. If your signs and symptoms get worse, you ought to appearance out for those caution signs. They consist of:

• If a fever, wheezing or headache will become worse or intense.

• If you increase speedy breathing, shortness of breath, or chest pains.

• If you cough up blood or in case your phlegm will become darkish or rusty-coloured.

• If you emerge as drowsy or confused.

• If a cough lasts for longer than 3-four weeks.

• If you've got repeated bouts of acute bronchitis.

• If every other symptom develops which you are involved approximately.

CHAPTER FOUR

How is a chest contamination diagnosed?

Your physician can be capable of make a analysis of a chest contamination via way of means of paying attention to your tale and inspecting you. They will ask approximately your signs and symptoms and the way you're feeling. They may additionally ask approximately your scientific records and that of your family. They can be inquisitive about whether or not you smoke, how a great deal and for the way lengthy.

The exam might also additionally consist of checking your temperature. Sometimes your physician will test how a great deal oxygen is circulating round your frame. This is completed with a small tool that sits at the quit of your finger. The physician will concentrate in your chest, so they will need you to raise or take off your top. If you need a chaperone in the course of the exam, the physician will set up one. If you've got bronchial allergies, they will ask you to test your height glide measurement.

Often no assessments are wished when you have contamination of the huge airlines (bronchi) in the lungs (acute bronchitis) and your signs and symptoms are slight. If your signs and symptoms are extra intense and also you want to visit medical institution then you could want to have the subsequent assessments:

• A chest X-ray can be taken to make certain of the analysis and to peer how horrific the contamination is.

• Blood assessments and phlegm (sputum) assessments can be taken to discover which germ (bacterium) is inflicting the severe lung contamination (pneumonia).

This facilitates to determine which antibiotic medicinal drug is fine to use. Sometimes the germ (bacterium) this is inflicting the pneumonia is proof against the primary antibiotic. A transfer to any other antibiotic is now and again wished.

How can a chest contamination be prevented?

There are measures you may take to assist save you chest contamination and to forestall the unfold of it to others. For instance, washing your palms often reduces the threat of germs moving into your machine.

You can by skip a chest contamination directly to others via coughing and sneezing. So when you have a chest contamination, it is essential to cowl your mouth while you cough or sneeze and to scrub your palms often. You ought to throw away used tissues immediately.

What reasons a chest contamination?

The sizeable majority of URTIs are resulting from viral infections. Your immune machine will combat those off with none assist inside some days. Because URTIs are resulting from viruses in preference to micro organism, antibiotics might not assist in any way. .

Respiratory tract infections

Sometimes an contamination in the top airlines can unfold deeper, inflicting a chest contamination. Sometimes germs (micro organism) already dwelling on your lungs can multiply, with the identical result.

There are primary varieties of chest contamination - acute bronchitis and pneumonia.

• Acute bronchitis - bronchitis is irritation   because   of contamination of the bronchi. is the scientific time period for irritation. It may be acute or continual. Acute approach lasting a quick time and continual approach lasting an extended time. Acute bronchitis is common and is frequently because of a viral contamination. Infection with a germ (bacterium) is a much less common purpose. See the separate leaflet known as Acute Bronchitis for extra details.

• Pneumonia - this is often a bacterial contamination of the lung and can be severe. Treatment with antibiotics is commonly wished. See the separate leaflet known as Pneumonia for extra details.

Who receives chest infections?

Chest infections are very common, mainly in the course of the fall and winter. They frequently arise after a chilly or flu. Anyone can get a chest contamination however they may be extra common in:

• Young kids and the elderly.

• People who smoke.

• Pregnant women.

• People with lengthy-time period chest troubles together with bronchial allergies, COPD, cystic fibrosis, coronary heart disorder, diabetes, kidney disorder or liver disorder.

• People with an immune machine it truly is weakened both via way of means of situations together with a few cancers (inclusive of lymphoma, myeloma and leukaemia) or AIDS; or via way of means of remedies together with excessive-dose steroids, chemotherapy or different drugs that may suppress your immune machine.

THE END

www.ingramcontent.com/pod-product-compliance
Lightning Source LLC
Chambersburg PA
CBHW070750260726
48660CB00007B/3049